COMPLETE BODY ALIGNMENT

Table of Contents

As result of modern day activities such as repetitive movements, and work or home related chronic postural strain, there is a tendency for the joints responsible for maintaining an ergonomic plumbline to become imbalanced. Included, are the weight bearing joints from the base of the skull to the ankles. Over time the insidious nature of biomechanical imbalances within the human body results in musculoskeletal pain and over time the possibility of joint irritation.

Entailed in this book is an effective way to realign the aforementioned joints to return them to an ergonomic balance. The effect of using these techniques, include relieving both joint irritation and muscular strain.

Contained in this literature are relatively simple manipulations which can be incorporated directly into currently used treatment techniques or employed entirely on their own.

The motivation for developing these techniques was the frustrating perpetuation of patient's physical disorders on subsequent clinic visits and the desire to improve results with treatment.

The underlying desire for writing this working manual was to simplify assessment and treatment techniques for other therapists and practitioners without being influenced by biased subjective pain complaints from patients. The end result, ultimately manifesting in improved treatment outcome.

ILIOLUMBAR ALIGNMENT

ALIGNMENT ASSESSMENT

This assessment technique is typically employed when the patient presents with lumbar pain. If there is hip pain with the lumbar complaint, it may possibly be a referred pain associated with a lumbar imbalance.

Figure 1

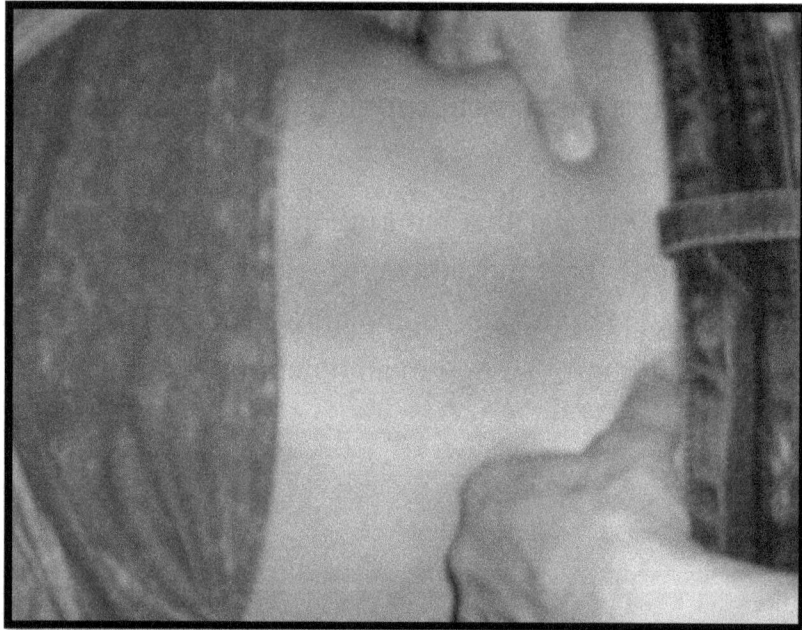

With the patient lying prone on the plinth, the therapist's index fingers are placed bilaterally pointed towards the floor on the patient's iliac crests. This is to visually measure the level of the iliac crests relative to the patient's spine. It will appear that one iliac crest rests lower than the opposite one relative to the patient's spine. The iliac crest which appears lower will typically, but not exclusively have pain in the area of that sacroiliac joint. It may also be apparent that the posterior superior iliac spine on the opposite side is rotated in an anterior fashion. This is a product of the body trying to maintain an ergonomic balance.

APPLIED ANATOMY

For any lumbar pain the quadratus lumborum muscle is inevitably involved. With palpation it will become apparent that the quadratus lumborum muscle will be hypertonic, increasingly on the depressed side than the elevated side.

Commonly, the iliopsoas on the depressed side will be hypertonic and when that occurs, the lumbar erector spinae on the opposite side will present with tension. This occurs as the body tries to maintain a balance.

In long term cases of misalignment, the presence of adhesions may be observed within the thoracolumbar fascia.

TREATMENT APPROACH

The muscles involved in treatment include hip flexors such as iliopsoas, rectus femoris and, sartorious. The abdominal obliques as trunk flexors also become involved. When aligning the iliac crests the above muscles are the major factors in activating the adjustment. The conscious participation of the patient is required.

Treatment begins by addressing the iliac crest which appears higher or, elevated superiorly. With the patient lying prone, the therapist places the anterior surface of their fingers just inferior the anterior superior iliac spine so as not to impart pressure on any bony surface.

Figure 2

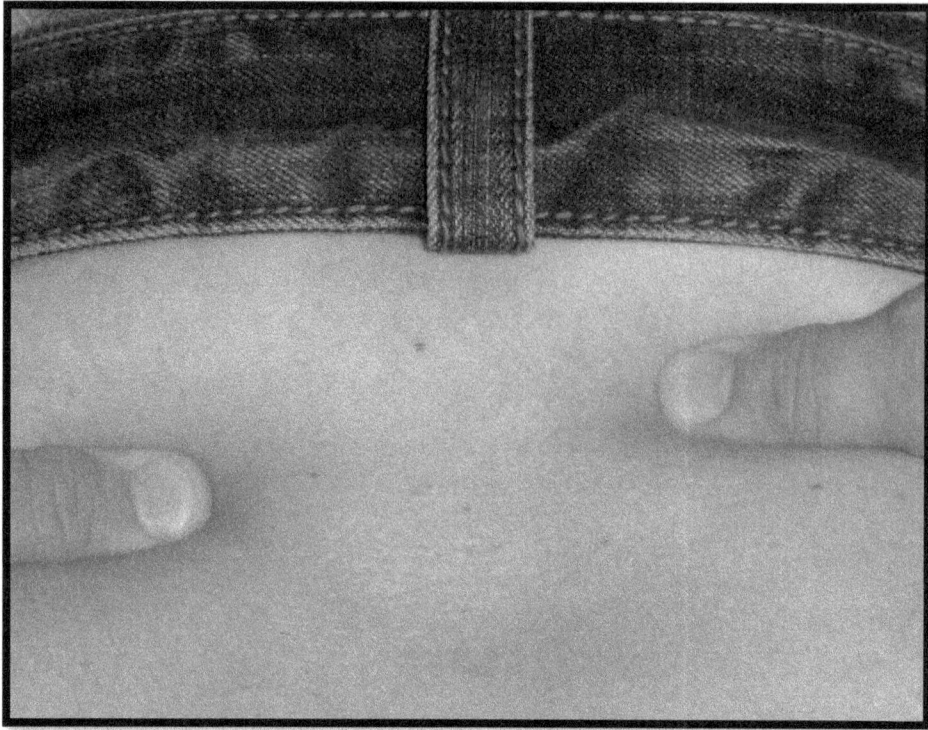

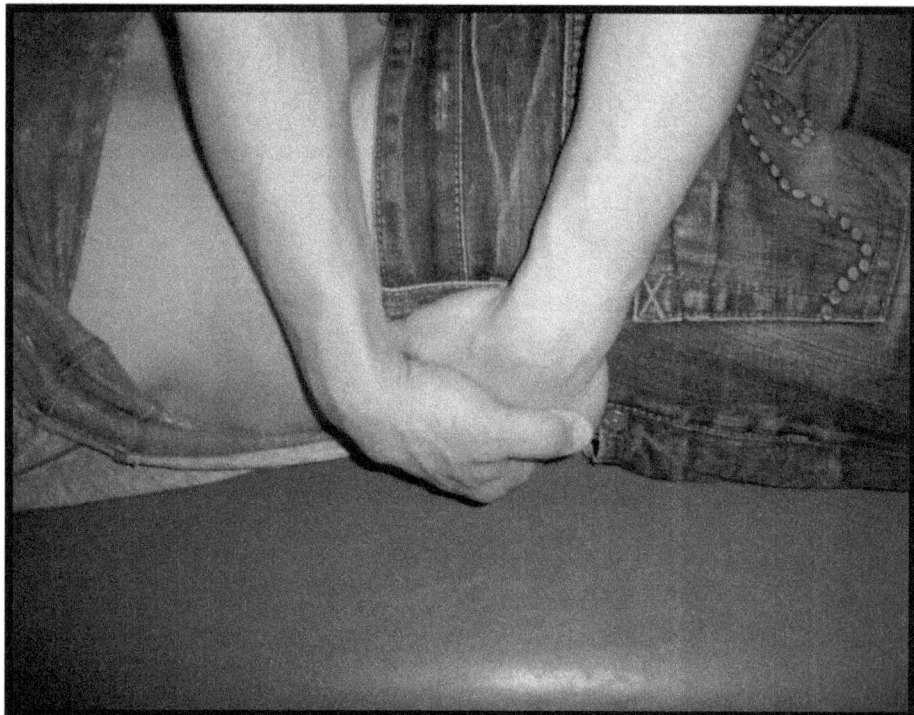

Care must also be taken not to create point digital pressure on the soft tissue. For the patients left side, the contact hand of the therapist is the left. For the patients right hip the therapist uses their right hand for contact. The therapists contact is maintained between the metacarpophalangeal joints and the distal interphalangeal joints. The contact hand may then be supported with the other hand.

Figure 3

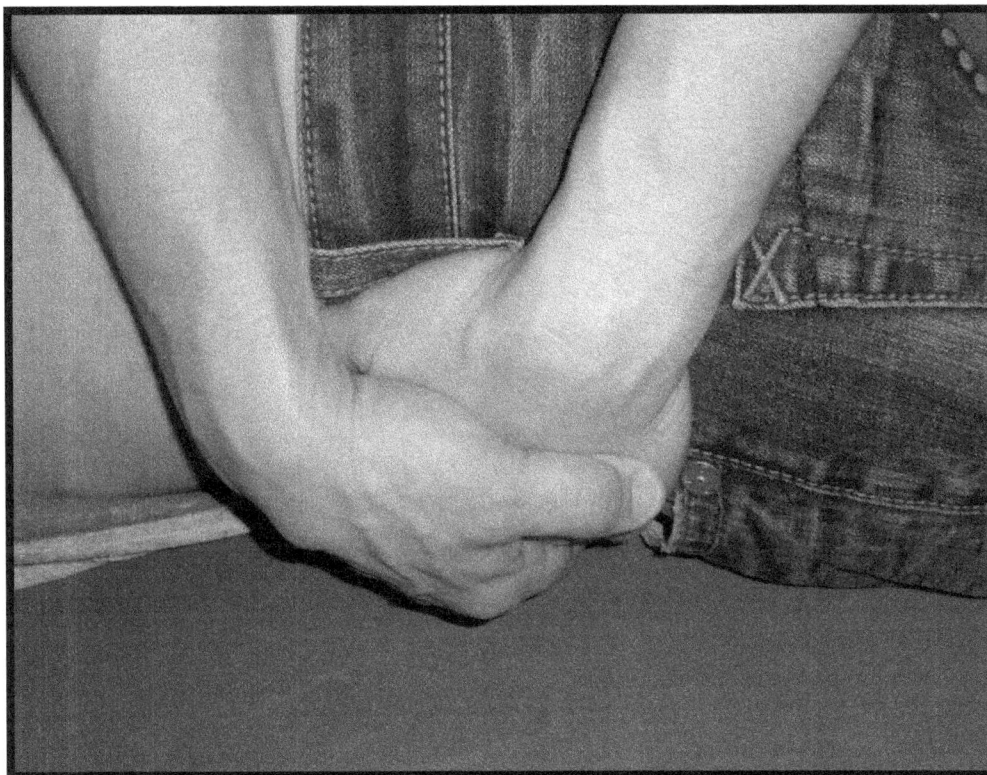

The therapist then creates a slight posterior rotational pressure on the patient's hip.

Care must now also be taken not to traction the skin as this may be quite uncomfortable for the patient as the procedure ensues.

The patient is then asked to create an anterior push at the hip for two to three seconds as the therapist resists any movement with an equivalent posterior draw. This resistance imparted by the therapist should inhibit any anterior movement of the patient's hip. The force exerted by the patient should not exceed one half of the patient's full strength, which will vary by the individual. When the patient pushes, they should not reach the point of pain.

Figure 4

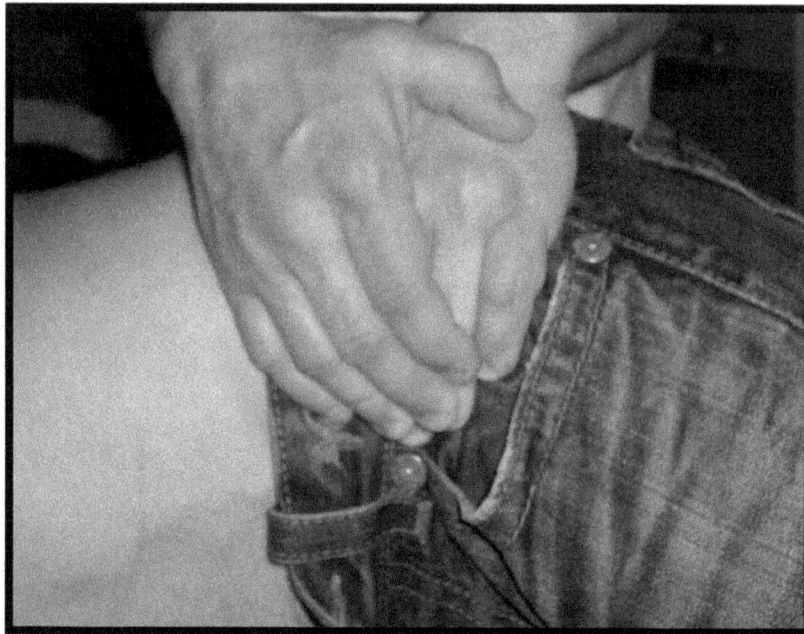

Following each compression the patient is asked to relax as the hip is lowered to the plinth. The hip is then rocked in order to find a "sticking point", where the body begins to resist further passive movement.

Figure 5

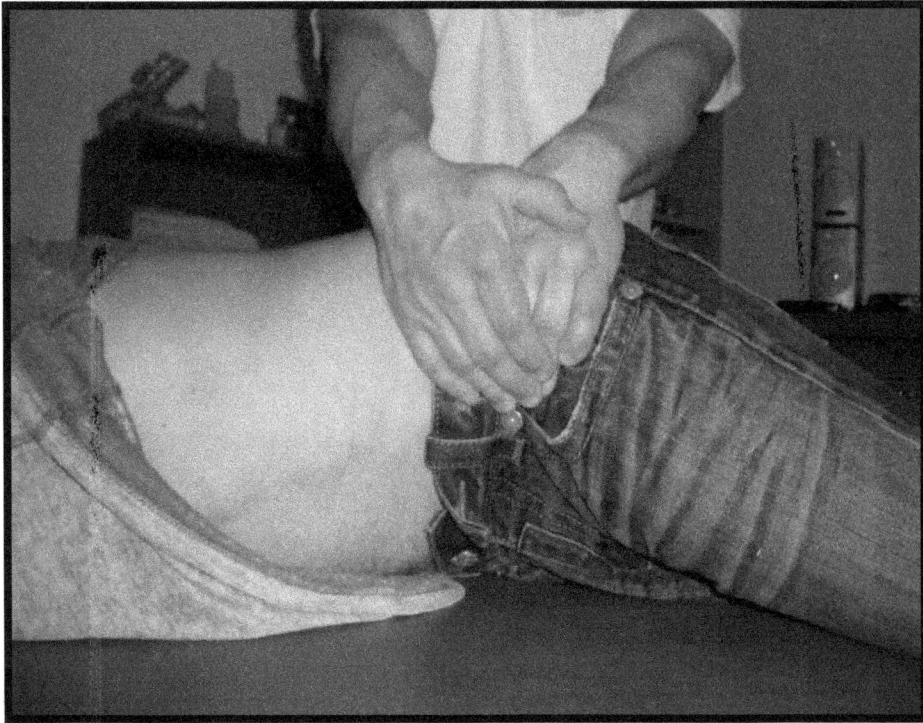

At the point where the body begins to resist passive movement, the same procedure is carried out where the therapist resists the anterior push of the patient. The patient is then asked to relax as the hip is lowered to the plinth and then passively rocked in an anteroposterior motion. With each compression cycle the therapist should be capable of moving the patient's hip further posteriorly before the next compression cycle. Each procedure is a compression cycle, where the resistance of the anterior push by the therapist is followed by a rocking motion of the patient's hip.

Following each set of three compression cycles a stretch ensues. This is performed by grasping the left hip in a similar manner as with the compression cycles. The left lumbar erector spinae are stripped cephelad.

Figure 6

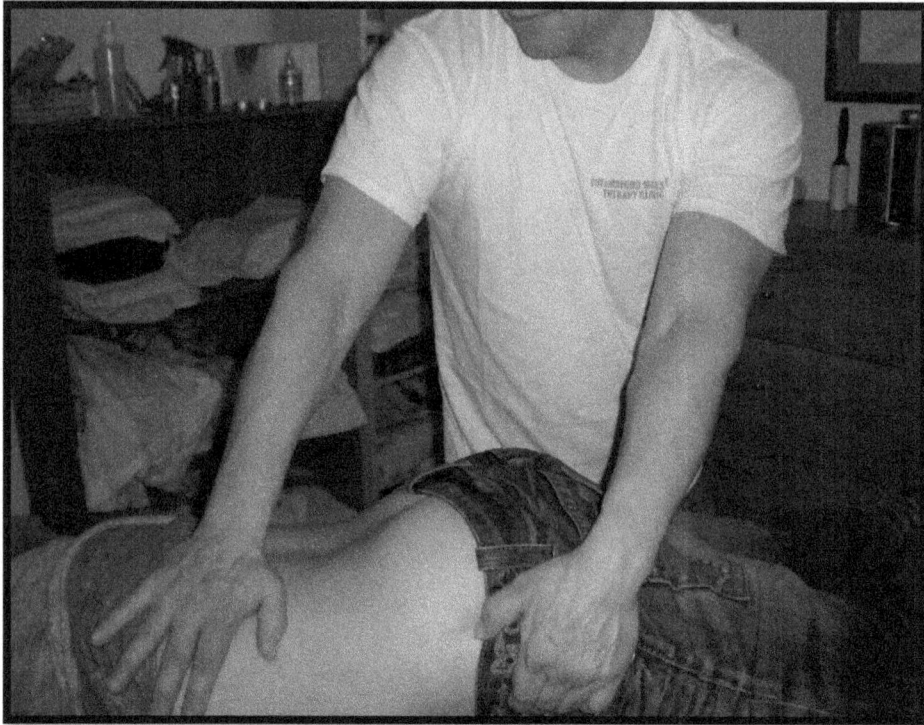

If this stretch is being performed without a lubricant, then stationary compression is performed with the right hand, as opposed to a glide which would be achieved with a couplant.

Figure 7

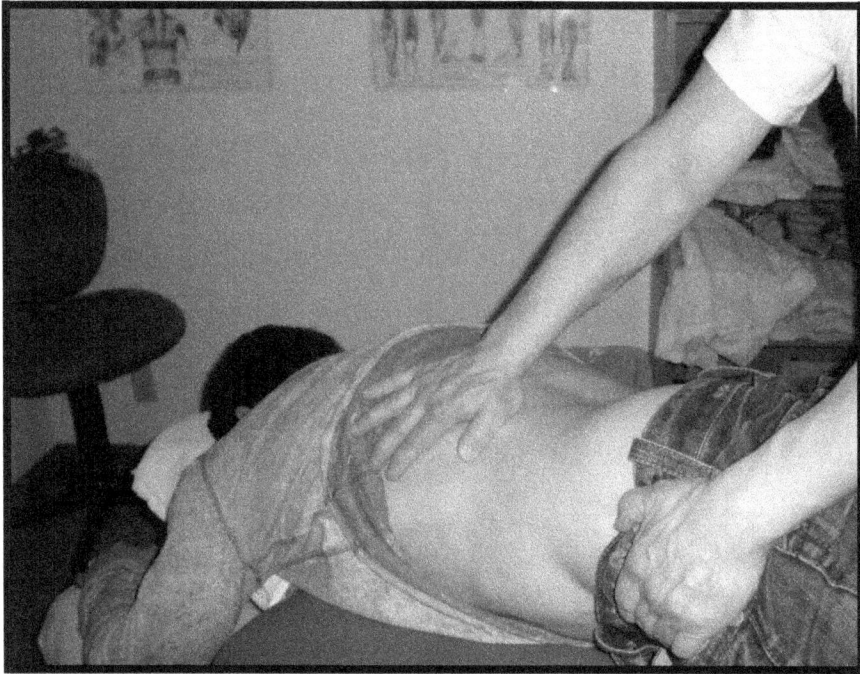

A traction accompanied by a torque is performed by creating an inferoposterior draw on the pelvis while the opposite hand creates a counteractive contact on the lumbar erector spinae on the same side. With each stretch, the hand in contact with the erector spinae moves superiorly to approximately the level of the 9th thoracic vertebrae. This stretch is performed up to three times per side. Care is taken to ensure that the patient does not begin to guard against the movement of the stretch.

Following three compression cycles and stretch, the therapist then performs the same procedure on the opposite hip.

Once the compressions and stretches have been performed the iliac crests are measured again to ensure that they are level.

PELVIC ALIGNMENT

ALIGNMENT ASSESSMENT

Following the alignment of the ilium, the alignment of the pelvis needs to be examined. Often there is a rotation in the pelvis which accompanies hip misalignment. This rotation of the pelvis will contribute to lumbar pain. This pain typically manifests in the area of the sacroiliac joint. This is caused by poor ergonomics often as a result of professions which require long periods in a sitting position. Another more in depth cause is protective muscle tension secondary to an underlying cause.

Assessment of alignment begins with the patient lying supine on the plinth. Leg lengths are measured at the medial malleoli for any discrepancy. It is not prudent to measure at the calcanei as there may be slight discrepancies as result of unilateral hypertension in the gastrocnemius and soleus muscles.

Figure 8

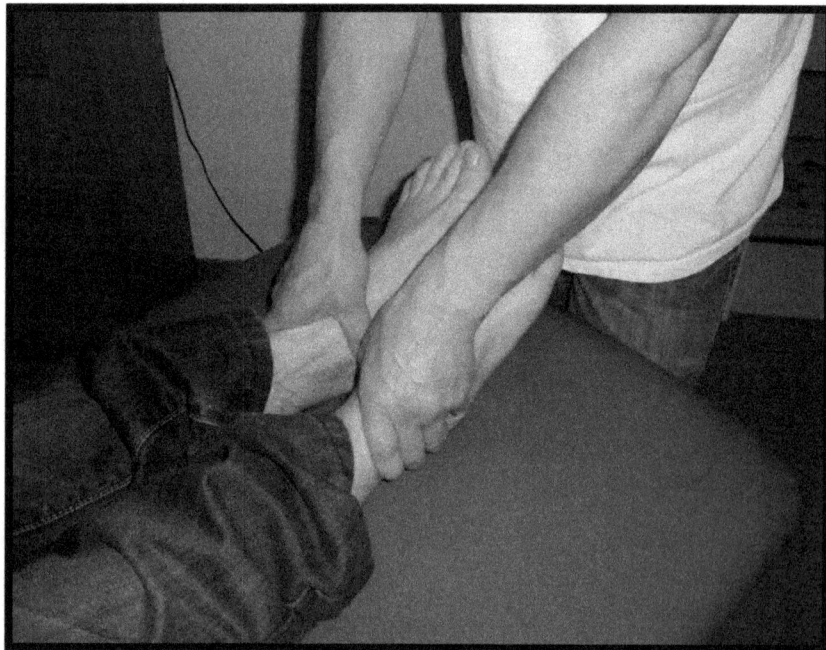

Figure 9

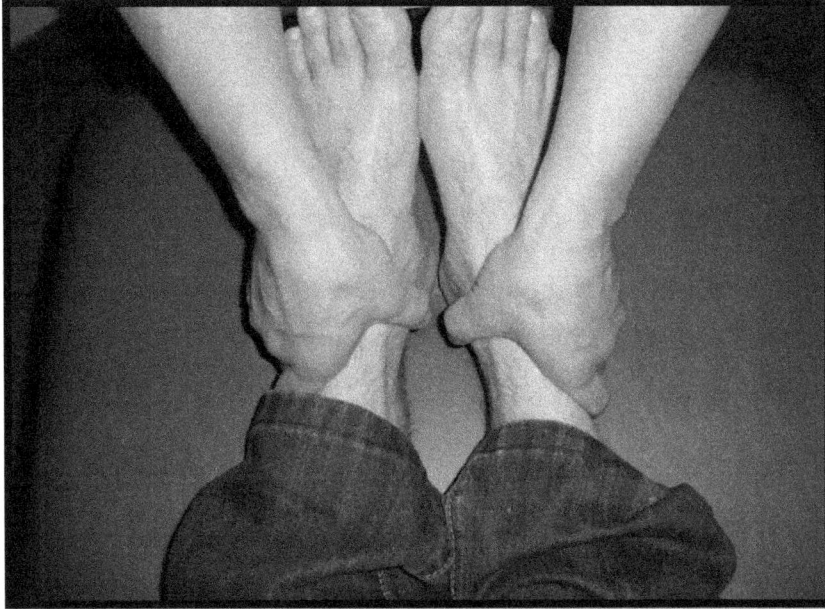

If one leg appears shorter than the other then a measurement of the pelvis at the anterior superior iliac spines is performed as a plumbline analysis.

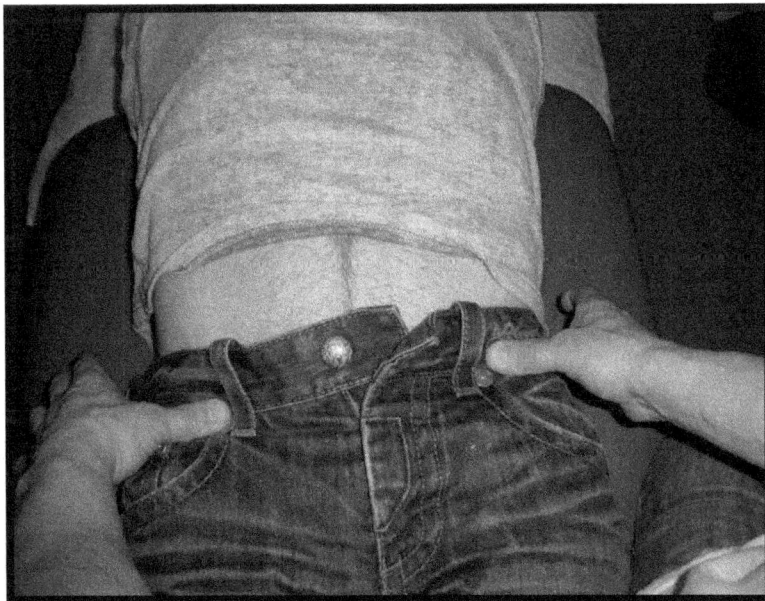

In the comparative analysis of the anterior superior iliac spines one will appear displaced inferiorly while the other is positioned superiorly relative to the plumbline. Typically the anterior superior iliac spine which appears higher is the side where the leg seems longer. There are, however, cases where the side which appears lower, will be the side where the leg appears longer. Nevertheless the superiorly displaced side is the one which is treated.

APPLIED ANATOMY

The muscles involved here are those which are involved with the iliolumbar area. Here the focus is more with the rectus femoris, tensor fascia lata and sartorious proximal attachments.

TREATMENT APPROACH

With the patient in a supine position, the hip and knee are flexed to ninety degrees with the foot planted on the plinth. The therapist then firmly yet gently grasps the ankle while the patient is asked to rest their knee against the therapist's thorax. The contact by the therapist at the patient's ankle is accomplished by supinating the hand and grasping superior to the malleoli. (Left hand for the left side). At the same time the therapist presses the thumb of their opposite hand into the tendinous attachments below the anterior superior iliac spine. Only a slight overpressure to surpass the surface tension of the tissues is required. The patient's hip is then flexed to raise the foot off the plinth. The hip is then further flexed and externally rotated until a muscular end feel is achieved. It is important that the patient remain relaxed and not assist in the movement of the hip. Any assistance by the patient will be palpable at the tendons being pressed as contraction of the tendon is palpated. It is important that the patient stay as relaxed as possible throughout the entire hip movement phase.

Figure 11

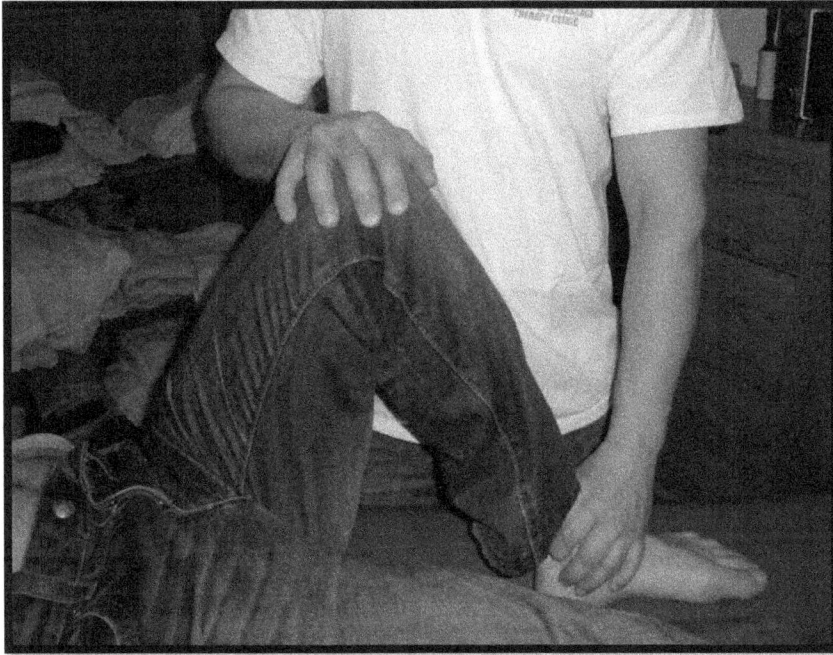

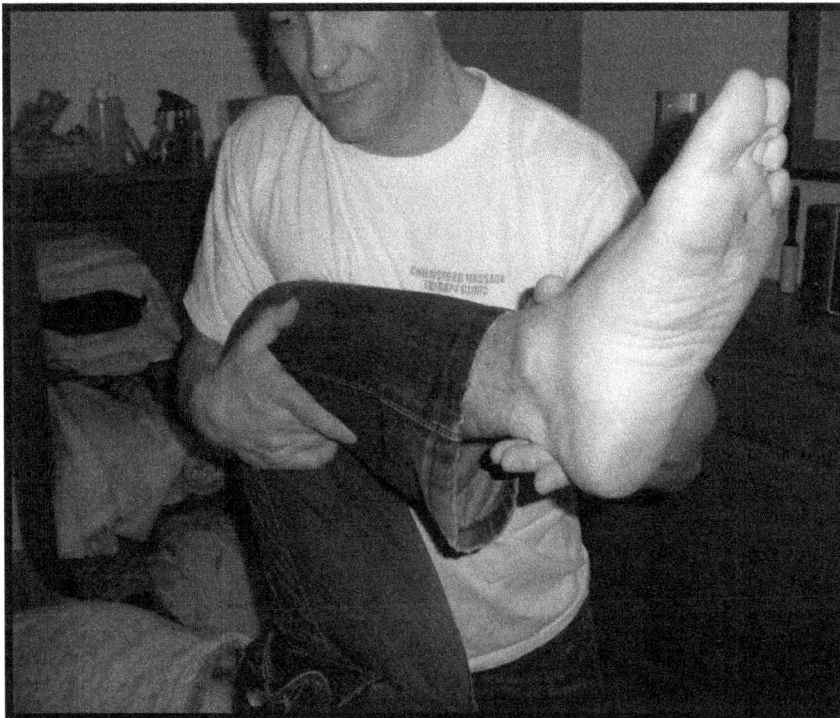

The patient's hip is then rotated back and, the hip and knee are extended back to the resting position on the plinth.

Figure 13

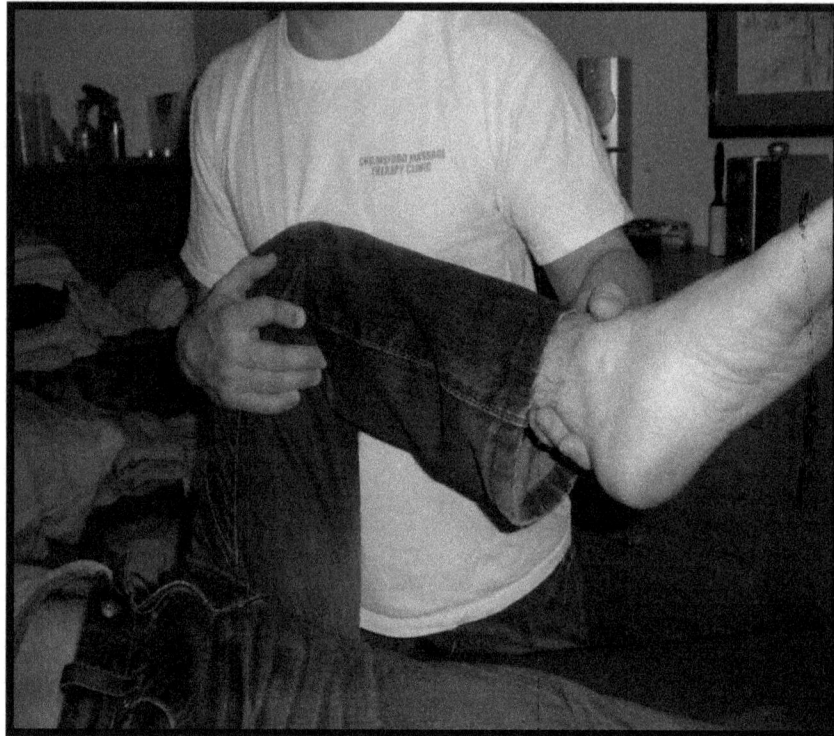

Following the return of the lower extremity back to the plinth, the anterior superior iliac spines are then re-measured to ensure that they are level. If the measurement still shows a discrepancy then the procedure is performed again. It is possible that the patient was guarding against the movement and that retarded the realignment. When the anterior superior iliac spines are level the malleoli are re-measured.

Following the alignment of the pelvis, the medial malleoli are measured again to ensure that they measure evenly. If there is a discrepancy, further measurements need to be performed to determine if a true leg length discrepancy exists.

It is possible that following the de-rotation of the pelvis and the inferior movement of the anterior superior iliac spine, that the opposite anterior superior iliac spine may seem elevated. If this is the case then the opposite side must also be de-rotated. The same procedure is followed for the opposite side to create an inferior movement of that anterior superior iliac spine. The pelvis is then measured again to ensure that it is level relative to the midline of the body.

ILIOPSOAS ASSESSMENT

To complete the pelvic alignment regimen one more assessment needs to be performed. This is done to ensure complete de-rotation of the pelvis.

With the patient lying supine, the therapist brings the patients arms above their head into full shoulder flexion with their palms facing anteriorly. The arms are then visually measured at the carpometacarpel joints of the first digit for a length discrepancy.

Figure 15

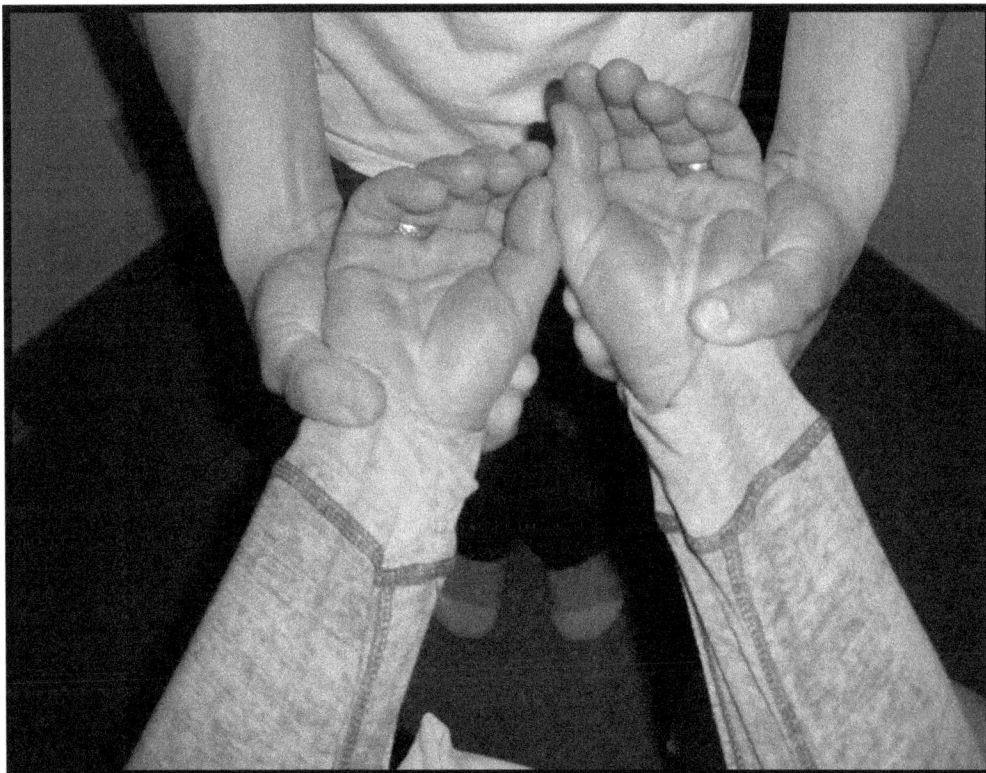

If one arm appears shorter than the other, then that is the side which has a contracted iliopsoas muscle. At that point an iliopsoas release must be performed to de-rotate the pelvis.

Following the release of the iliopsoas the arms are then measured again for a length discrepancy above the patients head. Again the most efficient measure of arm length is extrapolated from the proximity of the first carpometacarpal joints of each hand. Without inducing a great deal of manipulation discomfort around the injured area, a great deal of pain relief can be achieved for the lumbar area. If there was apparent glenohumeral stiffness upon performing the assessment, then that is often also relieved following the iliopsoas release.

This is not necessarily a permanent all inclusive resolution of the insulting factor causing the musculoskeletal dilemma, however, further orthopaedic assessment will be easier to apply. In many cases the condition improves dramatically within 24 hours, if immediate results are not obtained.

The factors which affect the desired pain relief are the chronic nature of the problem and the degree of irritation of the involved joints.

TREATMENT APPROACH

The most efficient way to release psoas is to flex the patient's hip and knee into a 90 degree position while they are lying supine. The halfway point between the umbilicus and the anterior superior iliac spine is measured. The patient then rests their knee against the therapist's

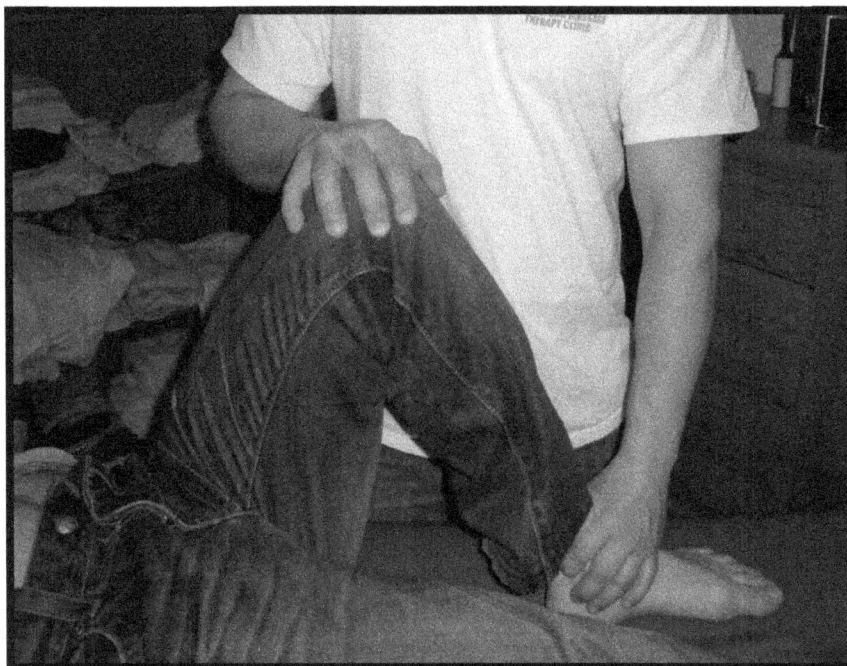

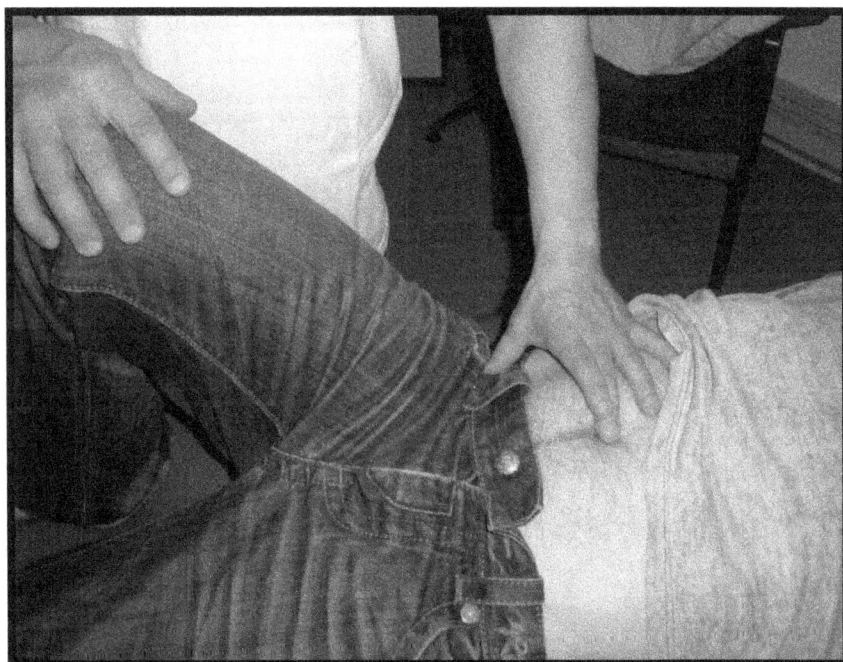

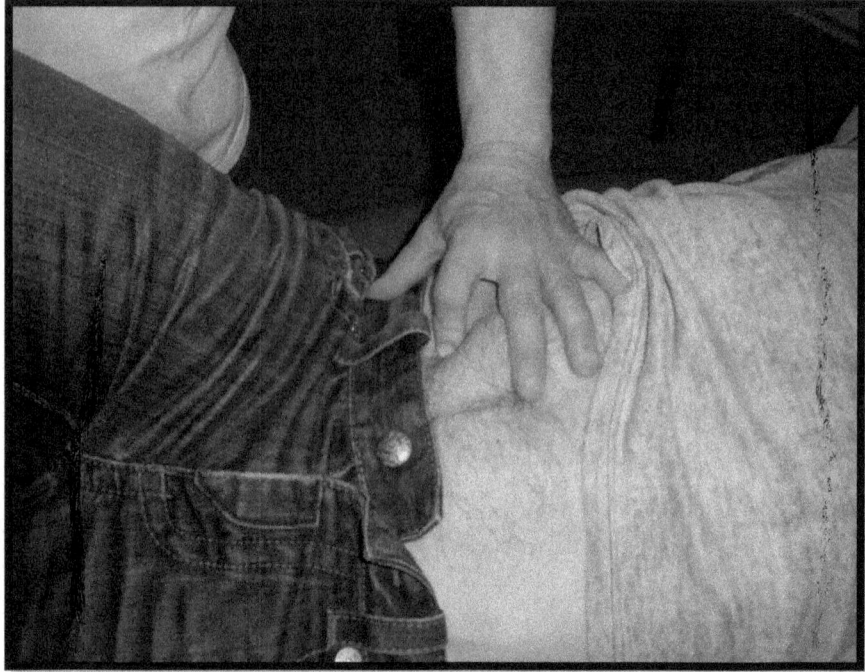

figure 2 1

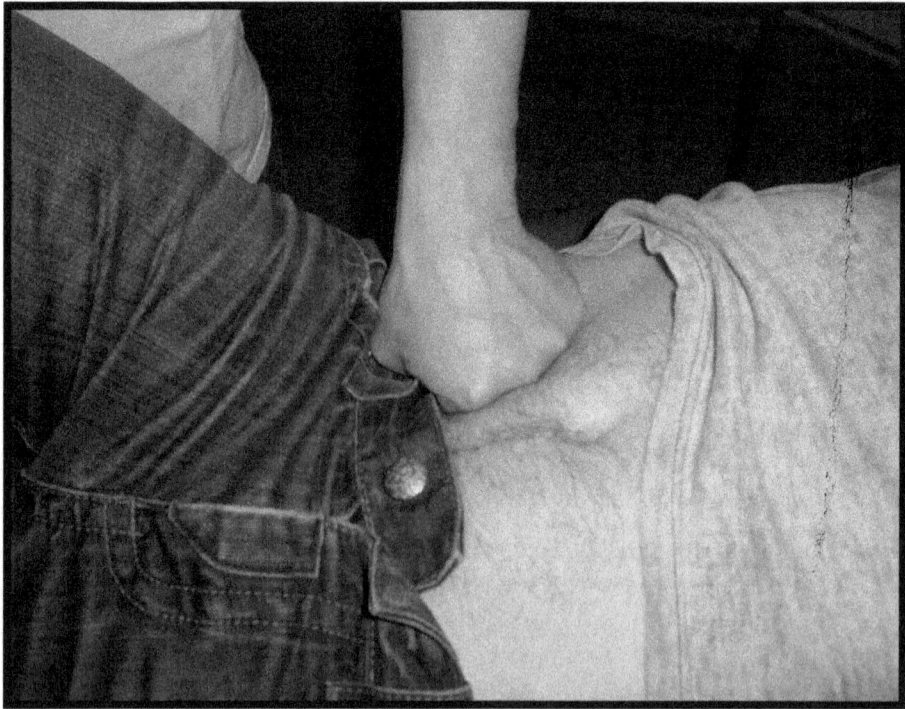

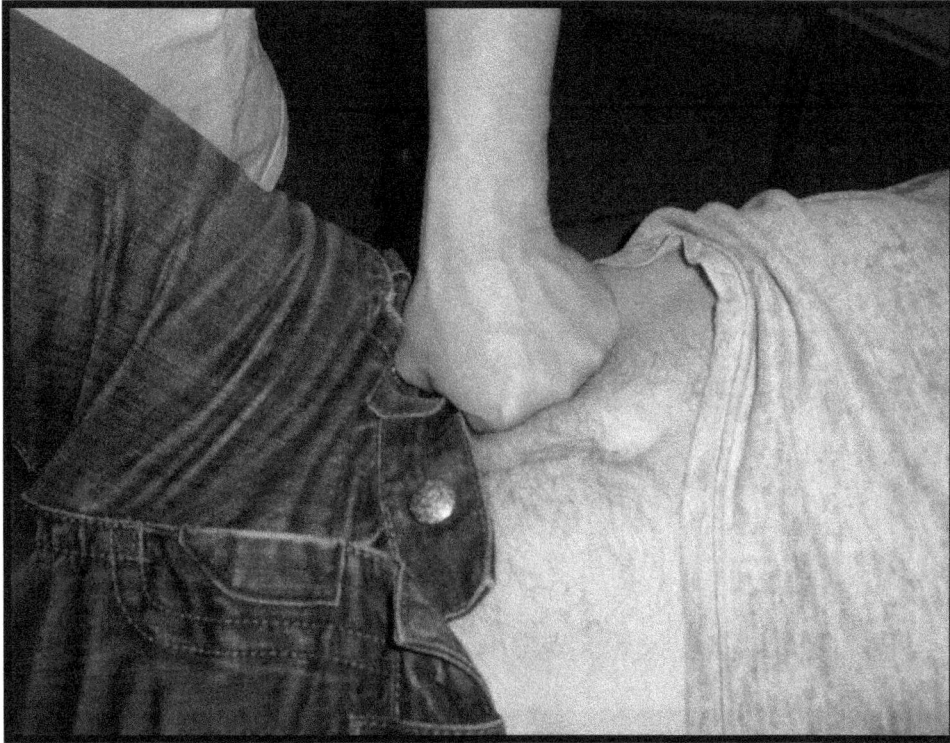

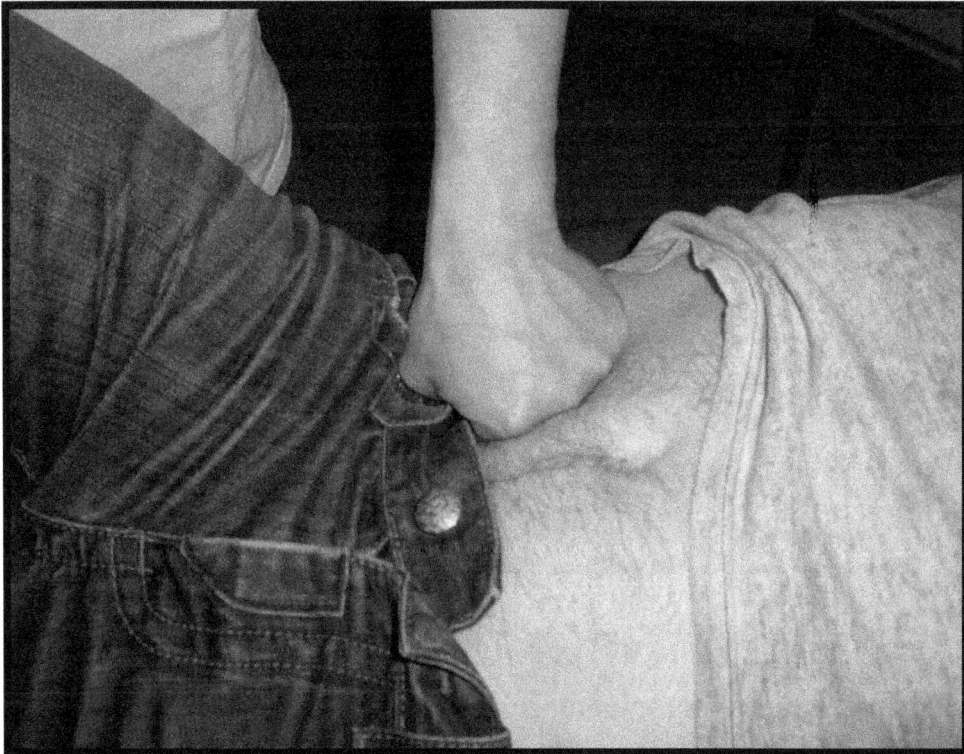

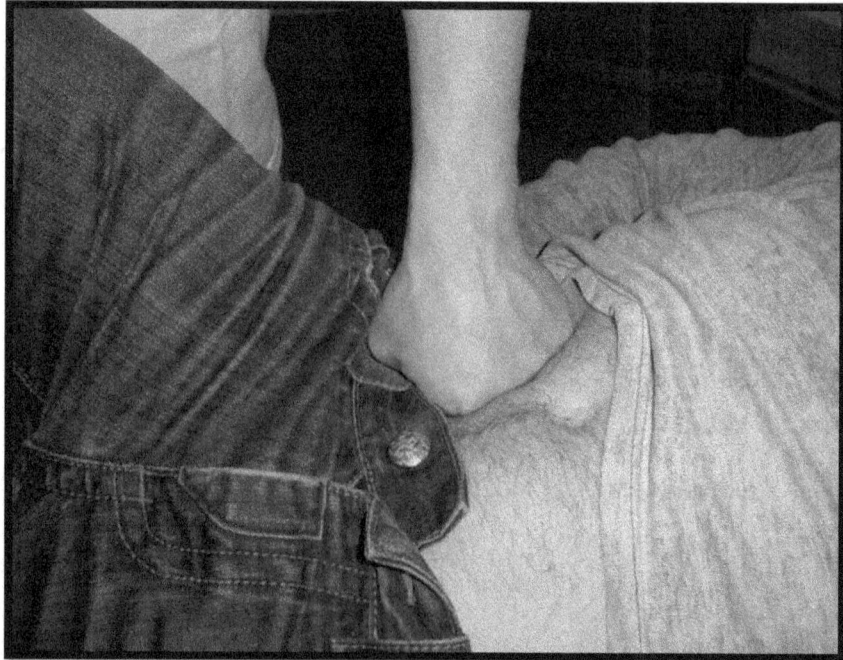

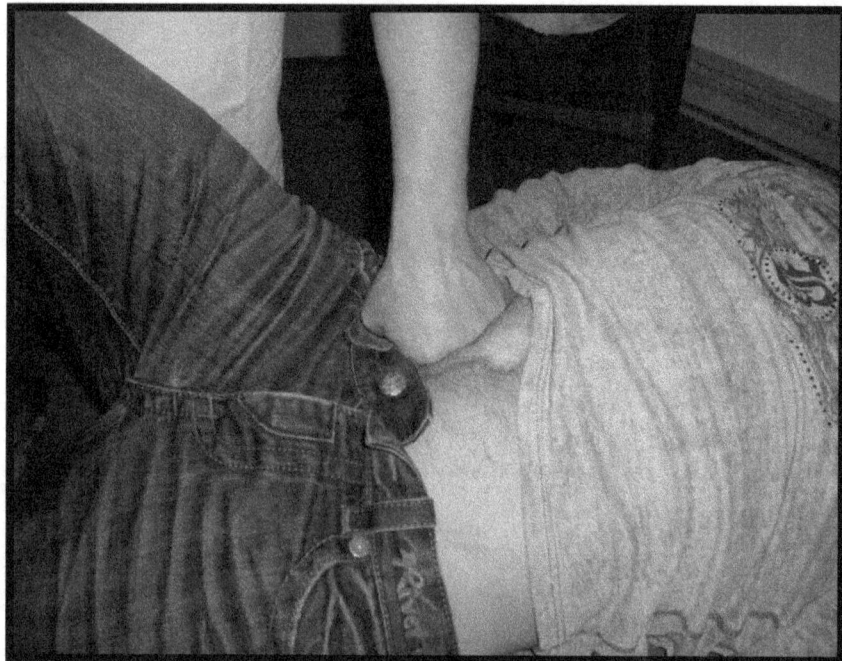

thorax and is instructed to completely relax the hip. The patient's foot is supported by the therapist's hand to prevent it from sliding down the plinth. The therapist then gently presses into the area over the psoas until it has released. At this point the hip and knee are extended back to the plinth and the arm lengths are measured.

THORACIC ALIGNMENT

ALIGNMENT ASSESSMENT

This manipulation is effective in relieving thoracic, sternal and, acromioclavicular pain. There is also significant pain inhibition in costosternal and costovertebral pain perception.

Beginning at the zyphoid process, the therapist glides their thumbs along the costal angles bilaterally to the bilateral notches along the 10th rib.

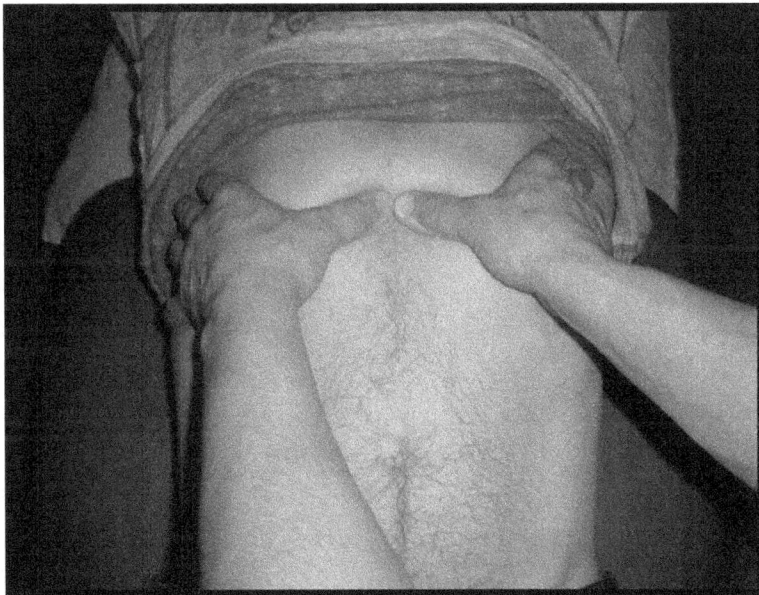

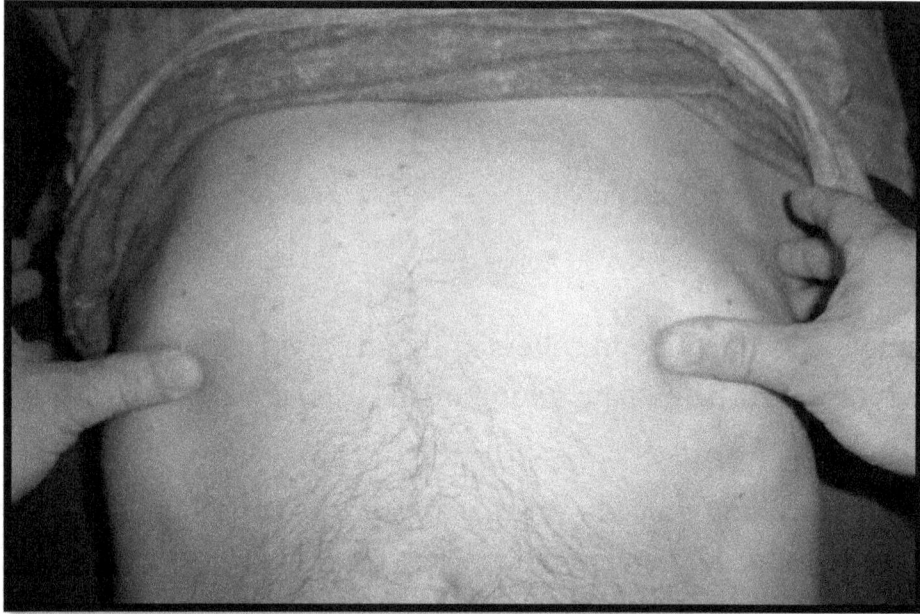

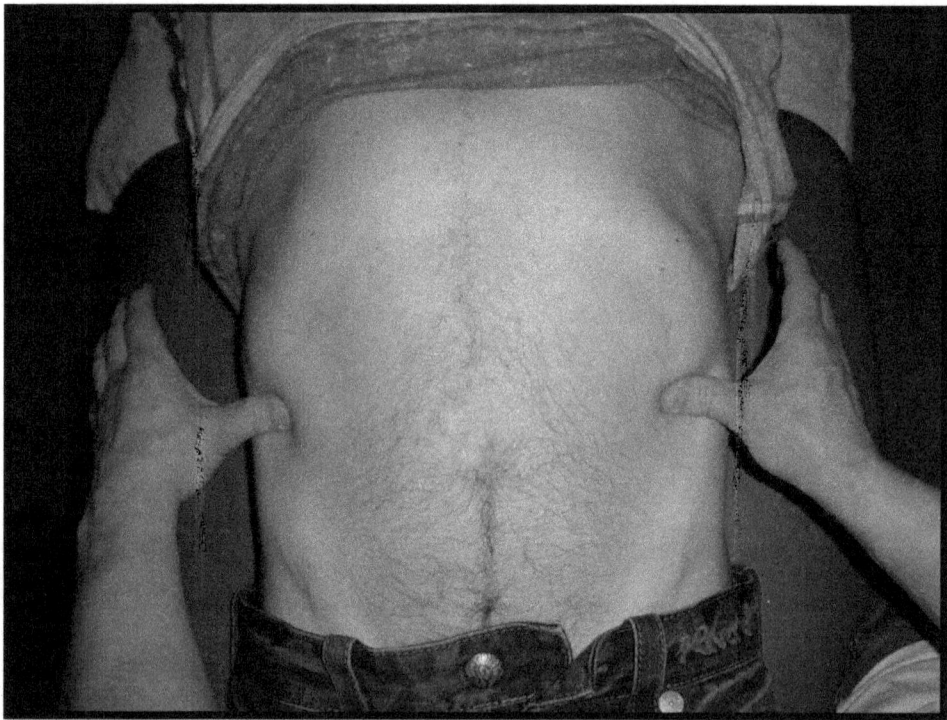

A plumbline measurement is then performed visually. With this measurement, one side of the thorax will appear inferiorly displaced relative to the opposite side. It typically is the inferior side which will present with the affliction. This will manifest as acromioclavicular pain, thoracic pain or, sternoclavicular pain.

TREATMENT APPROACH

With the patient supine on the plinth, treatment begins with addressing the inferiorly displaced side of the thorax first. The patient's hands should be tucked under their hips to allow the shoulders to be completely relaxed. It is important that the patient relax their shoulders so that the thoracic alignment may occur. It is also important to iterate this to them so that they are conscious of the requirement as an essential part of the manipulation.

The inferior hand is placed posterolaterally along the 10th-12th ribs (for the right side of the thorax, this would be the left hand) and the superior hand makes initial contact along the costal angle slightly inferior to the zyphoid process.

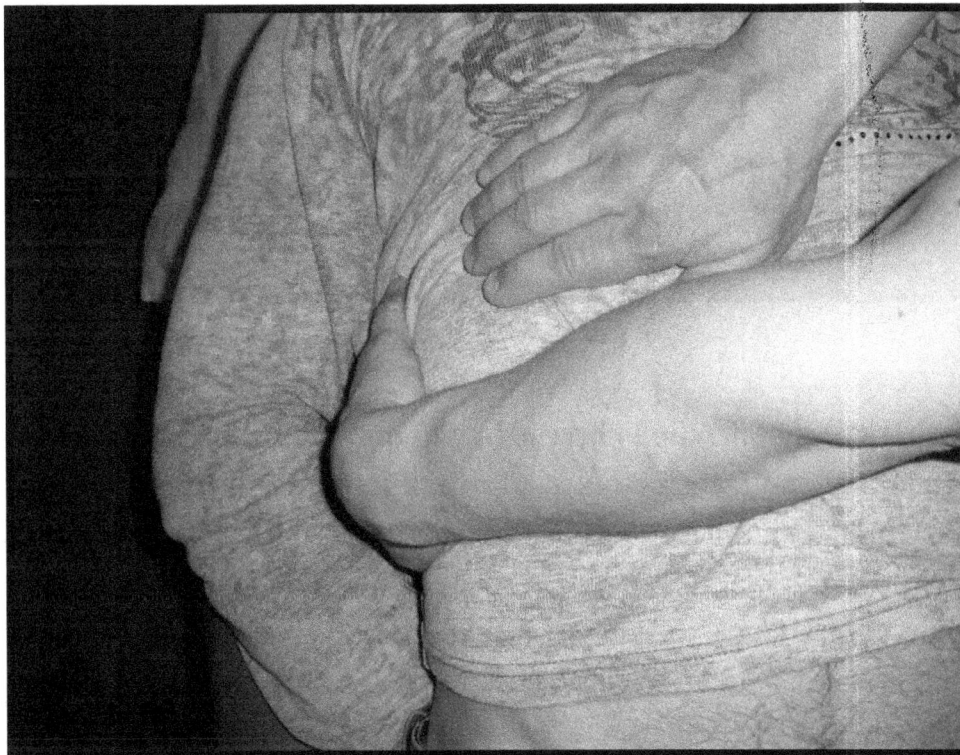

The contact of the superior hand is made with the thenar and hypothenar eminences. The thorax is then gently rotated in a posterior and anterior direction (rocked) using no more than 25-30 mm of Hg. The thorax may be rocked as many as eight times to achieve a smooth joint mobility and to allow the patient to fully relax. The superior hand is then moved a hand breadth cephelad slightly above the zyphoid rib process. The inferior hand is then advanced equidistantly in a cephalad direction to maintain mobilization of, and contact with the same ribs.

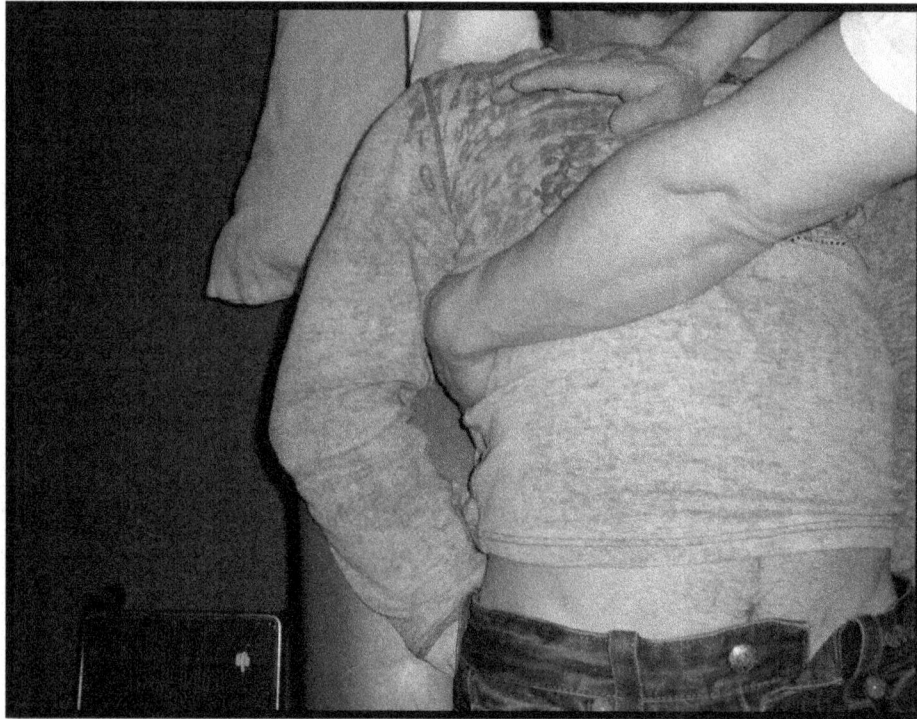

During the thoracic mobilization observe the fluidity of the movement as well as any atypical or unusual end feel. As this is a form of joint play all joint and bone health concerns and mobilization contraindications need to be considered to determine efficacy of the manipulation. With the patient's health history in mind, if there appears to be excessive rigidity in the thorax initially, the patient is encouraged to take a breath in and out and to relax their thorax and shoulders. On that note it should be reemphasized that the patient's shoulders need to be completely relaxed. If they are not, the costal shift (rib alignment) is unlikely to occur. The patient is encouraged to continue to breathe normally while the rocking motion continues.

The therapist then, in an uninterrupted motion, moves both hands continuously superiorly until the superior hand reaches the manubrium. If the right hand is the superior one, then the hypothenar eminence should make final manipulative contact at the sternal notch. The inferior hand will make contact on the ribs, anterior to the scapula as it comes to the completion of its superior movement. Then, the therapist performs the same manipulation in an inferior direction until the original starting point is reached.

Upon completion, the therapist then moves to the opposite side of the patient and proceeds with the identical mobilization on that side.

It is not atypical to encounter sensitivity at the costosternal joints of the patient. Factors include postural irritation of these joints, previous injury or, chronic inflammation. If there is costosternal irritation and sensitivity, therapist contact pressure needs to be decreased.

Upon completion of the thoracic mobilization, the level of the ribs is visually measured to ensure realignment.

If the thoracic alignment did not occur then the same manipulation is performed again with relaxation of the patient shoulders being reemphasized. Anxious anticipation resulting in contraction of shoulder musculature is the main deterrent in nonalignment. If, during mobilization in a relaxed state, the corrective shift does not occur, diaphragmatic release needs to be considered.

APLLIED ANATOMY

The structures involved include the ribs and their intercostals muscles. Also intimately involved are the vertebral facet joints and costosternal joints. With the mobilization there is also an effect on the costoclavicular joints and acromioclavicular joints. As the movement of the ribs occurs, the holding elements of the joints including the ligaments and joint capsules are encroached.

OCCIPITAL ALIGNMENT

This manipulation is quite interesting in how alignment is achieved. What I discovered and how this approach came about, was seeing an imbalance in the levels of my hands when performing cervical traction. These patients presented with headaches which were often previously diagnosed as common migraines. They also presented with hypertonic cervical spine muscles and often associated temporomandibular joint pain or dysfunction. Commonly there are sternocleidomastoid trigger points. It would behoove the therapist to determine the presence of coryza and/or the potential referral pattern of the headache.

ASSESSMENT APPROACH

This procedure is used to examine the occiput and its alignment relative to the cervical spine, with alignment emphasis on the joint relationship between the occiput and atlas. We should not exclude the axis, but for these purposes the focus should be on C0 and C1. This examination is efficacious in determining the prudence of occipital alignment for the treatment of headaches, cervical muscle hypertension and, cervical facet joint irritation. It may also be helpful in temporomandibular joint dysfunction.

With the patient supine on the plinth, the therapist approximates their index fingers to the mastoid processes of the temporal bones bilaterally while positioned at the head of the plinth. The therapist should be

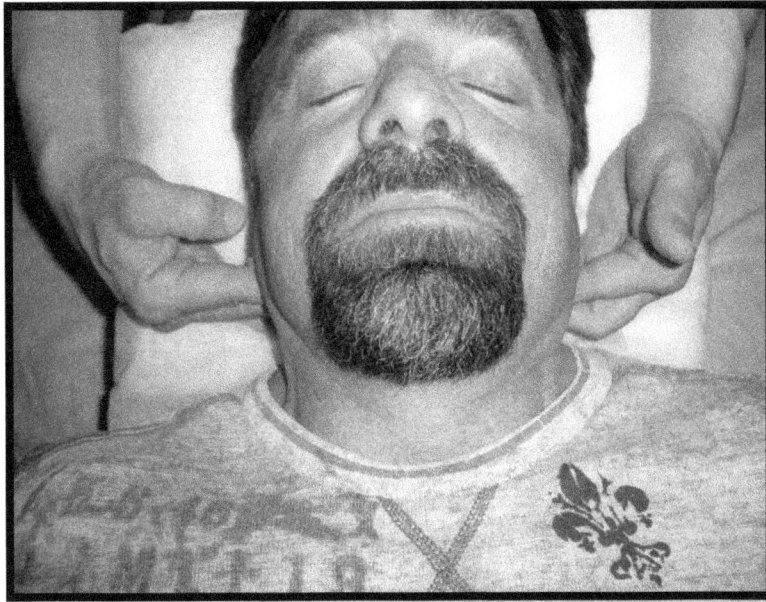

seated comfortably facing the patient to perform a visual plumbline assessment relative to the cervical spine. Both the index and third digit should be used to determine accurate land marking. The middle fingers are placed on the mastoid process bilaterally as the index fingers palpate the notch posterior to the external acoustic meatus. A visual examination of alignment then ensues to determine the direction of displacement. What will become apparent is that one mastoid process appears superiorly displaced while the other appears to be inferiorly positioned relative to the cervical spine.

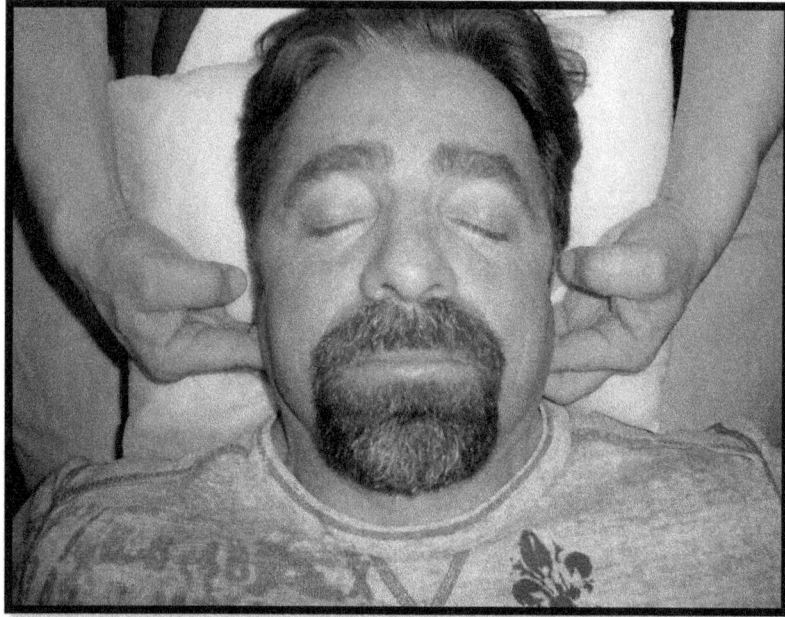

TREATMENT APPROACH

Upon determining the relative displacement of the mastoid process levels, the therapist approximates their hands to the lateral portions of the occipital and temporal bones in the area of the lambdoidal suture and squamosal suture.

At this point the therapist places the thenar and hypothenar eminences of their hand to create a rotational force for a vector translation along the sutures.

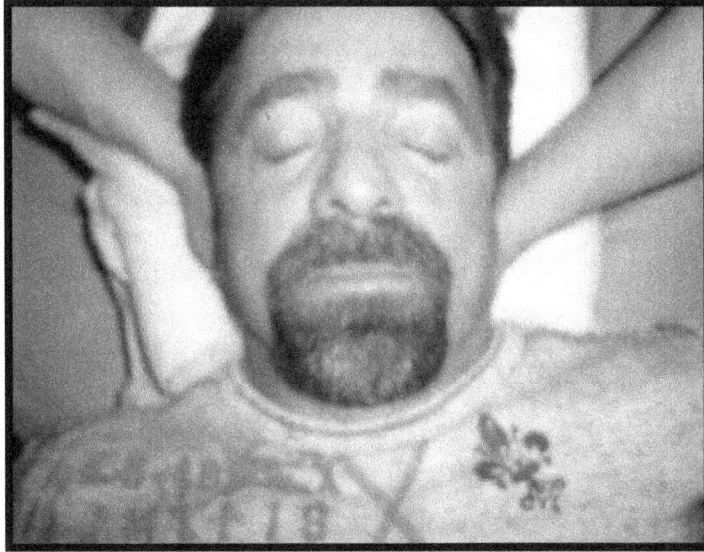

The inferiorly displaced mastoid process will encounter a supero-anterior rotational force from the therapist while the superiorly shifted mastoid process will be counteracted with an infero-posterior rotational pressure.

Only 15-30 mm of Hg pressure need be applied. As the therapist applies the rotational torque on the postero-lateral portion of the cranium, the patient is asked to open their jaw fully and hold it open for a count of three to five.

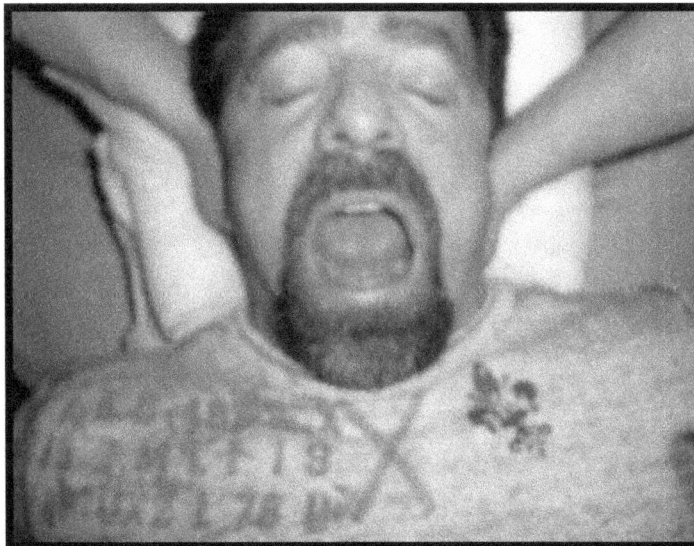

They must forcibly open their jaw as wide as possible to achieve the desired result of the cranial shift. There are quite often audible adjustments as the procedure is performed. Often where headaches are present, instantaneous relief of symptoms is achieved.

In cases of either prolonged occipital displacement or dramatic shifting prior to treatment, this procedure may need to be carried out as many as three times consecutively. In some cases if the procedure needs to be performed more than once, the patient may not be opening their jaw as widely as possible for fear of pain or inherent immobility. Following the three to five second translation, the patient is asked to close their jaw slowly. Emphasize that they are not to allow their jaw to snap shut. As elevation of the mandible occurs, observe any incongruency in movement.

Following each occipital alignment attempt, the mastoid processes must be examined to determine if alignment has been achieved.

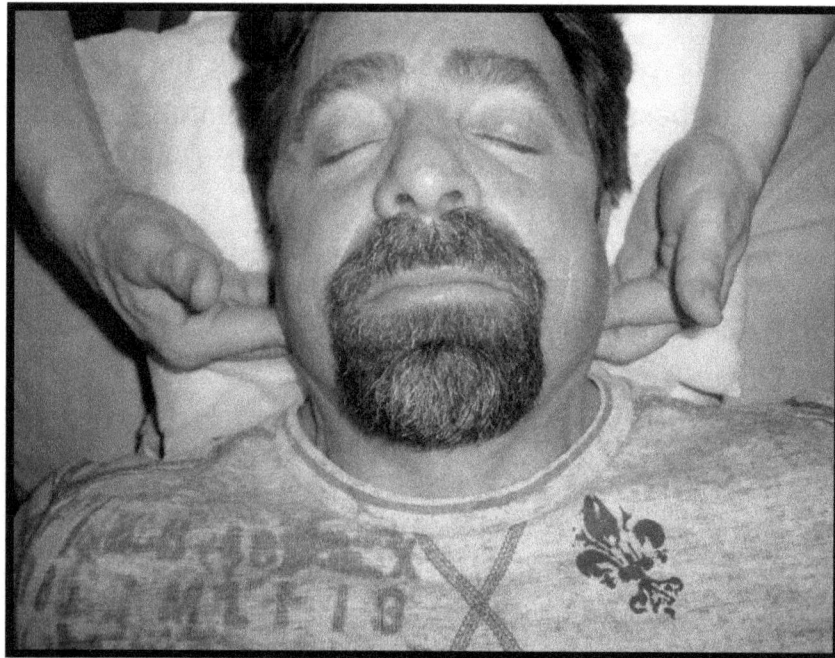

Once alignment of the occiput on the atlas has been accomplished a gentle traction may be applied to assist alignment through the entire cervical spine.

Cervical muscles should be palpated to ensure return to normal tension levels. If there is still a palpable hypertension then further manipulation or assessment may be required.

APPLIED ANATOMY

The stomatognathic system is involved with this manipulation. First of all, the sternocleidomastoid muscles by virtue of their attachment to the mastoid process as well as their function as the primary cervical spine flexor and rotator, can have a powerful effect on the misalignment of the occiput. Often these muscles are the referral source for headaches.

The atlas, the axis and, the occiput through their attachment with the suboccipital muscles are also involved in this manipulation and this occurs with the inherent extension of the cervical spine when forcibly depressing the mandible. This, however, does not exclude any of the other posterior cervical muscles involved in cervical spine extension.

The auscultation which can occur upon depression of the mandible is often the articular disc of the temporomandibular joint. This occipital manipulation can reduce the stresses placed on the articular disc reducing discomfort with depression and elevation of the mandible.

This concludes the description of the body alignment and is intended to dramatically improve the success of treatment irrelevant of your training and professional background. The success of treatment also improves with use of the techniques. Even with inherent patient inflexibility, success is dramatic.

ACKNOWLEDGEMENTS

I would genuinely like to thank Daniel McIntosh for being the model in the photographs and Maria McIntosh for being the photographer.

Sylvie Monette was instrumental in providing me with the technical computer assistance in designing the manual when I was at a loss. I am forever grateful to you all.

Mikael Kivi BA RMT

www.ingramcontent.com/pod-product-compliance
Lightning Source LLC
Chambersburg PA
CBHW081749200326
41597CB00024B/4450